GW00360100

Understanding

BACK PAIN

Professor Malcolm I.V. Jayson

Published by Family Doctor Publications Limited
in association with the British Medical Association

All rights reserved. No part of this publication may be reproduced, or stored in a retrieval system, or transmitted, in any form or by any means, electronic, mechanical, photocopying, recording and/or otherwise, without the prior written permission of the publishers. The right of Malcolm I.V. Jayson to be identified as the author of this work has been asserted in accordance with the Copyright, Designs and Patents Act 1988, Sections 77 and 78.

IMPORTANT

This book is not designed as a substitute for personal medical advice but as a supplement to that advice for the patient who wishes to understand more about his/her condition.

Before taking any form of treatment YOU SHOULD ALWAYS CONSULT YOUR MEDICAL PRACTITIONER

In particular (without limit) you should note that advances in medical science occur rapidly and some of the information contained in this booklet about drugs and treatment may very soon be out of date.

THIS IS THE JANUARY 1997 EDITION

© Family Doctor Publications 1997

Medical Editor: Dr Tony Smith
Consultant Editor: Lynne Low
Cover Artist: Colette Blanchard
Medical Artist: Angela Christie & Philip Wilson
Design: MPG Design, Blandford Forum, Dorset
Printing: Reflex Litho, Thetford, Norfolk, using acid-free paper

ISBN: 1 898205 31 0

Contents

Back problems can range from mild, occasional discomfort to continuous pain. For some people back pain is an occasional twinge, for others it can be disabling and agonising. Figures from the National Back Pain Association reveal that 80% of people with back pain suffer a recurrence and it is the second most frequent request doctors receive for help after the common cold.

When back pain is severe, no position is comfortable and all movements are painful, even coughing and sneezing. Pain in any form is a warning and back pain is often associated with the inflammation of an injured or misused back, so reducing inflammation is a vital part of pain control. In this case, the best choice of painkiller is one which will help control both pain and reduce inflammation.

Since it was launched as an over-the-counter breakthrough in pain relief, clinically proven **Nurofen** has been used by millions of pain sufferers to provide fast, effective relief from a wide range of painful conditions, such as back pain. **Nurofen 400** provides the same level of pain relief as two Nurofen tablets in a single tablet format. Alternatively, **Nurofen Micro-Granules** deliver all the pain relieving benefits of Nurofen in a fast-acting, soluble format. For powerful pain relief, try dual action **Nurofen Plus**, which contains the active ingredient in Nurofen with the additional power of codeine.

For a free Nurofen Guide to Backache, send a SAE (min 7" X 10") to Nurofen Backache Guide, PO Box 193, Nottingham NG3 2HA.

Alternatively the Nurofen Advisory Service runs a series of 24-hour automated telephone helplines designed to offer practical advice:
Battling With Back Pain – tips to get you back on your feet

0171 617 0815

Nurofen contains ibuprofen, always read the label.

Introduction

Backache is not an illness in itself, but a symptom. Its development means that something has gone wrong somewhere, although it may not always be clear exactly what.

Most of us suffer from backache at some time or other. Usually it is an unpleasant, awkward but not desperately serious problem caused by some kind of mechanical stress or damage within the back which gets better fairly quickly. Poor posture, excessive stresses, and wear and tear problems may be at least partly responsible.

You should not be surprised that backache is so common when you realise that your spine is composed of many different structures, including bones, discs, ligaments, tendons, nerves, blood vessels and other tissues, all of which can be affected by mechanical damage resulting in backache.

In most cases the precise cause of the problem is not important. Backache is a symptom which will clear up and the purpose of treatment is to relieve pain and to make sure that you recover as soon as possible. Occasionally there may be a more severe underlying cause and detailed investigations are required to decide the right approach to treatment. Understanding how the back works will help us to protect our spines and recover more rapidly from attacks of backache.

This booklet aims to show you how the back works, what goes wrong, why back problems arise, how they are treated and to give some indication of when further investigations and specialised help are necessary.

A GROWING PROBLEM

Backache is remarkably common. At any one time some 30 to 40 per cent of the population have backache and between 80 and 90 per cent experience it at some time in their lives. It affects both sexes and all ages from children to elderly people but is most prevalent in the middle years.

Backache is one of the most common reasons why people have to take time off work, especially in heavy manual industries. At particular risk are workers in the building industry and nurses who often have to undertake heavy lifts in awkward postures.

It's often hard to separate cause and effect: in other words, do the stresses in the job cause the backache, or is the person unable to do heavy work because they already have a bad back? In many cases, back pain follows some injury or a sudden twist. Much time is

Back pain on lifting.

WHAT PATIENTS SAY

Back pain can take many forms, but the following complaints are typical:

'I work in a factory assembling components. By the end of the day I have a terrible aching pain low down in my back and I really don't know how much longer I can stand it.'

'I am not too bad during the day but I wake up in the morning with a lot of pain and stiffness in my back and have to get up and move around before it eases.'

'I bent over to pick up a book from the floor and felt a sudden severe pain in the bottom of my back and couldn't straighten up.'

'While I was working in the garden I got a twinge of pain in my lower back. Over the next few hours the pain spread into my bottom and down the back of my leg. It has really hurt and I have had to go to bed.'

now spent training workers to avoid subjecting their backs to excessive stresses.

The amount of working time lost due to back problems has increased enormously in recent years. It is now running at some 100,000,000 working days per year in England and Wales, two or three times more than 20 years ago. In fact, this dramatic rise does not mean that more people are being injured at work. Rather, it reflects the more concerned approach taken by both workers and employers to the effects of back pain. The result is a dramatic escal-ation in the costs of back pain to our society. This is now calculated as nearly £6,000,000,000 per year for the medical treatment provided, the benefits received and loss of production – a phenomenal sum.

The increase in the numbers of people disabled by back problems has led to a complete rethink of our approach to back pain and how it is treated. In this booklet I will provide the most up-to-date views based on the latest research on the treatment of back pain and explain how we are attempting to reduce the frequency and severity of this problem.

KEY POINTS

✓ Backache is a symptom not a disease

✓ Acute episodes of back pain, although unpleasant, usually get better quickly

✓ Backache affects 80–90 per cent of the population at some time in their lives

How your spine works

The spine or back bone is known medically as the vertebral column. Its role is to support the whole body, be capable of bending and twisting in all directions and at the same time protect the vital structures such as nerves which run through it. What's more, it has to last a lifetime. No engineering structure comes anywhere near meeting such specifications and it is hardly surprising that problems can arise from time to time.

THE VERTEBRAL COLUMN

Vertebrae

The human spine consists of a column of bony blocks known as vertebrae which sit one on top of another to form the vertebral column. There are seven cervical vertebrae in the neck, twelve dorsal or thoracic vertebrae in the upper and middle back, and five lumbar vertebrae in the lower part of the spine. The fifth lumbar vertebra is known as L5 and sits on the sacrum which in turn is connected to the coccyx – the tail bone. The sacrum consists of several vertebrae which have joined together. The sacrum is joined at its edges to the pelvis – the ring of bone which carries the trunk and which in turn is supported by the hips.

- **Discs:** The spine is not a rigid structure. It is able to bend and twist because there are flexible cushions or discs between each of the vertebrae. Each disc is a flat biscuit-shaped structure with a jelly-like centre called the nucleus and an extremely strong outer skin called the annulus.

- **Facet joints:** The vertebrae are also joined to each other by pairs of small joints which lie at the back of the spine, one on either side. They

Cervical vertebrae

Thoracic vertebrae

Lumbar vertebrae

Sacrum

Coccyx

Pelvis

The human spine showing cervical vertebrae in the neck, the thoracic verte▌

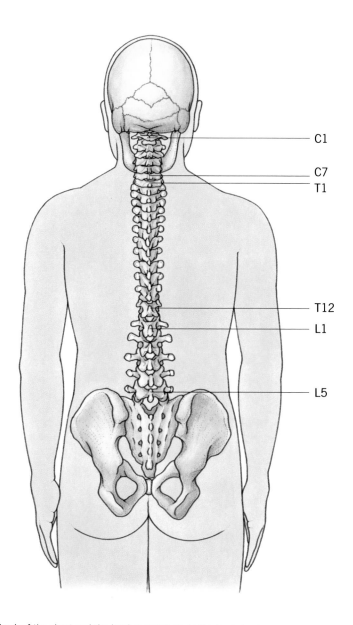

C1

C7
T1

T12
L1

L5

he back of the chest and the lumbar vertebrae in the lower back.

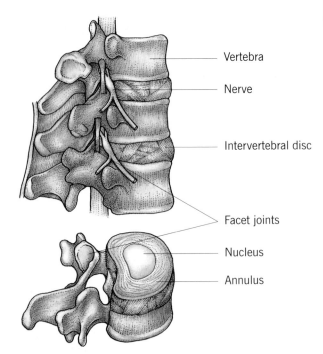

Vertebra

Nerve

Intervertebral disc

Facet joints

Nucleus

Annulus

Three vertebrae with the intervertebral discs in between and the nerves emerging from the sides. The disc at the bottom is shown in more detail with the inner nucleus and outer annulus.

can be affected by strain or by wear and tear and may develop bony swellings causing pressure on nerves.

• **Network of nerves:** The nervous system in some ways resembles a telephone network that carries messages from your brain to various parts of your body and back again. Messages that pass down nerves make muscles contract and so control movements such as walking. Those travelling up nerves carry sensations which eventually reach your brain so you experience sensations such as touch and pain.

• **The spinal cord and nerves:** A 'cable' of nervous tissue, known as the spinal cord, extends from the brain down the spine inside the canal formed by the vertebrae. The nerve roots divide off from the spinal cord, run for short distances within the canal itself and emerge in pairs, one on each side from the sides of the vertebral column to supply the body, the arms and the legs.

What happens in back injuries

The fact that the spinal cord carries messages to and from the body means that, if it is damaged, the 'connection' may be affected, which can lead to the loss or alteration of sensation, development of pain and weakness of movements. This is what happens when people become paralysed after a serious accident.

The number of limbs paralysed, i.e. whether they can move their arms and not their legs, or whether all four limbs are paralysed, depends on where the spinal cord has been damaged. If the injury is in the neck, paralysis and loss of sensation can affect both the arms and the legs. However, if the injury is in the thoracic or lumbar segments – below the arm level – then only leg muscles are affected. Fortunately most back problems damage the nerves but usually not the spinal cord.

Pain can therefore develop in the back itself resulting from direct injuries to ligaments, tendons, joints and other structures, and also because the same nerves that supply these tissues also supply the legs, with the result that patients may feel the pain as if it is arising from the legs. In addition, there may be pressure directly on the nerves, also producing pain, alteration in the sense of feeling and weakness in the legs.

It is clear that the back is a very complicated structure. When there has been some injury back pain may arise for several different reasons. Very careful analysis would be necessary to determine what has happened in any individual. Fortunately, most acute episodes of back pain get better without the need for specific forms of intervention.

As a result very detailed tests to determine the particular injuries causing problems are generally not required. However, when symptoms are more serious and prolonged it becomes important to determine exactly what is going wrong. Very careful examination and diagnostic tests, including some of the newer forms of imaging, may then become necessary.

KEY POINTS

✓ The vertebral column consists of vertebrae joined by discs and facet joints. The disc has a jelly-like central nucleus and an extremely strong outer skin, the annulus

✓ Pain may arise from damage to a wide variety of structures

✓ The pain is transmitted by the nerves. The ways that these are stimulated are complex and depend upon the particular tissue or type of nerve that has been affected

✓ As most acute episodes of back pain get better quickly there is no need for very detailed tests to determine the precise cause

Some common back problems

Now we know the make-up of the spine, it is easier to understand where and why problems can arise.

NON-SPECIFIC BACK PAIN

Many people who have trouble with their backs experience brief episodes of pain from which they make a full recovery. No firm diagnosis is made and so their back pain is called non-specific. Detailed investigations are not necessary and often it is not possible to identify the particular underlying cause. Sometimes the person has tender areas over the spine or between the sacrum and the iliac bone of the pelvis. The pain may be caused by strains of ligaments, tendons or other soft tissues.

Although the cause is usually uncertain, terms that imply that your doctor has actually made a diagnosis – such as lumbosacral strain and sacroiliac strain – are

often used. The term 'non-specific back pain' is preferable as it does not suggest that we know the cause of your particular problem. Further investigation to pinpoint the cause is only necessary if the back pain fails to settle.

DISCS – SLIPPED OR BURST?

Most people have heard of a 'slipped disc' but it is a rather inaccurate name because discs actually cannot slip. They can wear, split or burst. What happens is that, after some stress on the spine – often involving bending, twisting or lifting – the disc bursts or prolapses and the jelly-like central nucleus is squeezed out through a split in the outer annulus.

We now believe that most discs that prolapse in this way previously had some wear and tear changes and the stress on the spine then triggered the problem. In fact, the

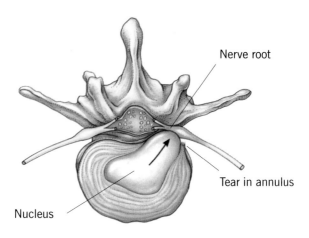

A disc that has burst backwards and to the side, pressing on the nerve root.

Nerve root

Tear in annulus

Nucleus

disc was already abnormal and would have burst sooner or later anyway. The particular stress probably just acted as a 'final straw'.

The jelly-like material, having been squeezed out, presses on the nerve running next to the disc causing severe pain in the back that spreads down the leg and sometimes as far as the foot. You may feel numbness and tingling, particularly in your lower leg and foot. Some of your muscles may become weak and the ankle jerk reflex, tested by tapping your Achilles tendon with a tendon hammer, may be lost. The site of these changes helps the doctor to identify exactly which nerve has been damaged.

The pain caused by a burst disc can be very severe. Usually the symptoms will slowly get better and eventually disappear completely. However, once the disc has burst it is permanently weak and there is always the risk of a further bout of back pain.

SCIATICA

As the greatest weight and bending forces are experienced in the lower part of the lumbar spine, the nerves most often damaged are the fifth lumbar nerve root, which leaves the spine between the fourth and fifth lumbar vertebrae, and the first sacral root, which leaves the spine between the fifth lumbar vertebra and the first part of the sacrum. These two nerves join together to form the sciatic nerve which runs down the back of the leg to the foot. Pain arising because of damage to this nerve is known as sciatica.

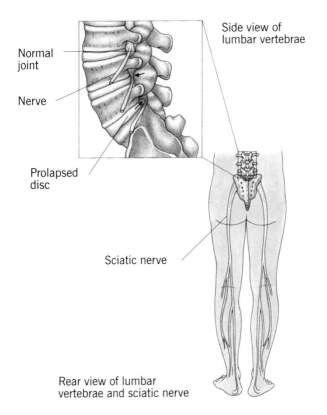

Side view of lumbar vertebrae

Normal joint

Nerve

Prolapsed disc

Sciatic nerve

Rear view of lumbar vertebrae and sciatic nerve

A burst of the L5/S1 disc pressing on the nerve root which forms part of the sciatic nerve travelling down the leg.

WEAR AND TEAR – SPONDYLOSIS

Spondylosis, or wear and tear of the spine, is very common. Indeed these changes start at about the age of 25 and are present in almost all of us by the time we are middle-aged. This is one of the main reasons why athletes are at the peak of their performance in their early twenties.

The lower back bears the weight of your whole body as well as anything that you're carrying, and does most of the bending and twisting. This is why wear and tear changes of the spine are most common in the lumbar region, and are called lumbar spondylosis.

Lumbar spondylosis is most likely to occur at the lower levels, particularly between the fourth and

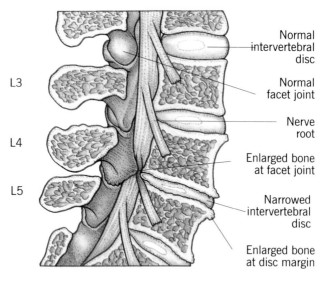

Enlarged bone at the margins of the facet joint and the discs pressing on the nerves.

Normal intervertebral disc

Normal facet joint

Nerve root

Enlarged bone at facet joint

Narrowed intervertebral disc

Enlarged bone at disc margin

L3

L4

L5

fifth lumbar vertebrae (L4/L5) and the fifth lumbar vertebra and the first segment of the sacrum (L5/S1), and leads to sciatica (see above). It affects both the discs and the facet joints. Some material is lost from the disc and from the cartilage or gristle lining the facet joints. The bone at the margins of the discs and facet joints enlarges, making movement more limited and so stiffening the spine. It may press on nerves, ligaments and other structures causing pain.

However, this is not as depressing as it sounds. The fact that you have these wear and tear changes does not mean that you are bound to get backache. Many people

have quite severe wear and tear changes with few or no problems, whereas others with relatively minor changes suffer incapacitating bouts of pain. It follows that wear and tear changes of this sort are generally of only minor significance.

LUMBAGO

One of the most common back problems is recurrent spells of acute pain which may spread to the buttocks or one or other thigh. While the attack lasts, your back may feel stiff and tender as well. When the symptoms are very severe the condition is called lumbago. The pain can last a day or

Normal nerve

Nerve trapped by
swollen facet joint

Nerve trapped
by prolapsed
intervertebral disc

The nerves may be trapped and damaged by the bony swelling.

two or up to a couple of weeks each time. Sometimes it then disappears completely or it may persist or recur. The symptoms are made worse by poor posture and heavy lifting.

X-rays frequently show the presence of lumbar spondylosis but surveys have revealed that these changes are often found in people who don't have any symptoms. It is therefore difficult to assess the part they have played in causing pain. Because of this, the term 'non-specific back pain' is often used to describe lumbago.

NERVE PROBLEMS

Nerves easily get squashed within the vertebral canal and as they emerge from the sides of the vertebral column by damaged discs, facet joints or vertebrae. When a nerve is squashed its ability to pass messages is affected. When this happens, you may experience pain or a sensation of numbness or tingling in the area supplied by the nerve, and the muscles it controls in your leg or foot may become weak. The spinal cord transmits these sensations to the brain – it is a bit like interference on a telephone wire, producing unpleasant noises and poor quality sound. In fact, current research indicates that it is a lot more complicated than that. Changes within the spinal cord itself can affect the pain message. This may explain why some patients continue to experience widespread and prolonged symptoms when the original nerve damage has healed and there is little evidence of much wrong with the back.

COCCYDYNIA

This is the name given to pain at the tail end of the spine or the coccyx. Usually no cause is found. A soft cushion ring may be used to make sitting more comfortable, but the condition usually settles by itself with time.

PROBLEMS WITH THE NECK

This section will deal only briefly with common neck disorders. The neck shares the same basic structure as the rest of the spine, and is therefore also prone to disc problems and wear and tear changes.

While pain in the lower back commonly shoots down the legs, neck pain may involve the shoulders and arms. For uncomplicated neck problems, treatment with rest, painkillers and perhaps physiotherapy usually suffice. A padded neck collar is helpful to ensure the

Neck collar.

neck is properly supported and rested.

Acute stiff neck syndrome
Many people have had the experience of waking up with a stiff and painful neck, often it seems for no particular reason. Movement may only be possible in one direction and the muscles of the lower neck may be tender. There are no other problems with the rest of the back or the arms or legs. The pain is associated with muscle spasm and will settle with a collar and painkillers in three to four days. Occasionally very gentle neck traction may help.

Whiplash
This is common after a car accident, when the sudden impact gives no time for muscles to brace, and the

Sudden deceleration
as when hitting a
vehicle in front

Sudden acceleration
as when your your car is
hit from behind

Whiplash injury to the neck in a motor vehicle accident.

head moves like a pendulum on the neck. In the simplest cases only ligaments in the neck are sprained, and the pain and stiffness that result are caused by the neck muscles going into spasm as a protective mechanism. If there are no other problems, a soft collar, pain relief and occasionally physiotherapy are all that are needed. In some cases pain persists for longer than six weeks, and it may be that the initial injury was more serious, causing damage to the discs or other structures, and has led to nerves being damaged or trapped. More detailed investigation is needed. Treatment may involve surgery. When pain remains severe for several months, it becomes more likely there will be continuing disability.

Disc problems in the neck

Discs can also prolapse in the neck, although this is less common than in the lower back. The neck is extremely stiff, and pain may shoot down one arm. Strength, sensation and reflexes in the arm may be lost. In the majority of cases, the pain will settle with rest, pain relief, traction if necessary, and then a period of gentle activation with a collar. Physiotherapy to strengthen the neck muscles is also useful.

Wear and tear problems

These changes are extremely common in the neck, and are known as cervical spondylosis. They may cause no problems at all, or lead to neck pain with headache and/or arm pain. Neck movements are reduced, and some patients have a tender spot in the trapezius muscle which lies between the neck and the shoulders. Again, the arms may become weak and lose their reflexes. There may be tingling or pins and needles in the arms.

In the most serious cases, the distorted bone and ligaments can press on the spinal cord affecting control of the arms and legs or an artery in the region, called the vertebral artery. This leads to dizziness, a buzzing in the ear and pain behind the eyes.

Many people who have cervical spondylosis also have low back pain. The principles of treatment are the same: rest in a collar, physiotherapy, anti-inflammatory drugs and pain relief. Surgery may be necessary for a small proportion of patients.

KEY POINTS

✓ Discs do not slip but they can burst

✓ Sciatica is caused by damage to either of the two nerves which join to form the sciatic nerve running down the lower limb

✓ Wear and tear or spondylosis on the spine is very common as you get older and correlates poorly with backache

✓ Neck problems have many similarities to back pain

Treating back pain – the first steps

Most of us get sudden episodes of pain in the back from time to time, usually lasting only a day or so. Apart from being careful you don't need to do anything about it and it is soon forgotten. Some people, however, may develop more severe attacks of pain which limit their activity and their ability to work.

Despite all our modern technology, in many cases we are not able to determine the exact source of the problem. It could well be the result of some damage to the ligaments, muscles or other soft tissues, but often your doctor may be unable to determine the precise cause. The good news, however, is that generally it does not matter as most of these acute attacks of back pain will get better rapidly.

The most common problem is simple backache in which the pain is confined to the back or may spread into the buttock or upper thigh. Sometimes it may extend right down the leg affecting the sciatic nerve, giving rise to sciatica. Pressure on this nerve may come from a damaged disc or other structures, causing pain and sometimes numbness and tingling running down your leg. Sciatica suggests that there has been some nerve damage and that recovery is likely to be slow.

Occasionally, a person may develop more severe symptoms which means that they need to be seen quickly by a specialist. This will be necessary for anyone who experiences any problems controlling the bladder or bowel, any numbness in the groin or rectal area or severe leg weakness, as it could be a sign of more severe nerve damage.

Details of the complaint are all important.

ASSESSING THE PROBLEM

Usually, when you have an acute back problem, the person treating you will ask for details about how and when the pain started and what has happened since, and give you a physical examination. Questions you may be asked include:

- Is the pain in one area or is it more general?
- Does the pain shoot or spread anywhere, e.g. the leg?
- How did it come on – suddenly or gradually? If gradually, over what period of time?
- Was the onset associated with any activity?
- Does anything make the pain worse?
- What is the pain like first thing in the morning?
- Are you otherwise well? Have you lost weight/got a cough/ other problems?

A pain which started on lifting a heavy object is sharp and limited to a small area, and is easier with rest; sleep is likely to be uncomplicated and the pain should get better rapidly. However, if the pain began gradually over many months, does not seem to be linked with movement, is becoming more severe and there are other problems such as weight loss, the cause may be more serious, and special investigations may be necessary.

When examining your back, the doctor may:

- Look for signs of curvature, and observe the way that it bends and how you walk.
- Feel your back for tender spots or areas.
- Perform the straight leg-raising test. The doctor lifts each leg straight up, when you are lying flat on your back. If there is a problem with the sciatic nerve, this will bring on the pain.

Examining the back.

The straight leg-raising test.

- Perform the femoral stretch test. The doctor places you lying on your front, then slowly bends each knee in turn. If there is a problem with another nerve called the femoral nerve, this will bring on the pain.
- Look for loss of sensation or weakness in the legs.
- Check your reflexes.

Testing the ankle reflex.

You may be sent for an X-ray, but usually this is not necessary. Although it may well show that you have some wear and tear changes, these features are common in people without backache and so don't have much influence on the choice of treatment. Each X-ray exposes you to radiation, which is why they should be reserved for people with severe back pain which has not responded to simple treatment and for those who have more complicated back problems.

You are unlikely to need more detailed types of imaging such as computed tomography (CT) or magnetic resonance imaging (MRI) scans.

TREATMENT

For most people with acute backache only very simple treatment is needed:

- Simple pain-relieving tablets such as paracetamol or ibuprofen. These tablets have few side effects and are usually all you'll need. You can ask your doctor for stronger painkillers which are available on prescription if you feel that you need them.
- A short period of bedrest is helpful, but too much can actually aggravate the problems. If you're in severe pain, you should rest lying flat in bed for a couple of days. After that, you can start to move around again, taking care to protect your back, but aiming to return towards normal physical activity.
- A cold pack – such as a bag of ice or frozen peas – against your back may help to relieve the pain. Alternatively, you can try heat in the form of a heating pad or a hot shower. However, neither is likely to make any long-term difference.

For most people, simple remedies such as these are enough and the pain will usually clear within a few days or a couple of weeks. You should aim to get back to normal physical activity as soon as possible. It is important that you take note of the advice in the chapter on how to protect your back so as to reduce your chances of having another attack in the future (page 25).

You may, however, be one of the unlucky ones whose pain does not disappear completely. If you still have a problem after about four to six weeks, you need to see a therapist. This might be:

- a doctor with special expertise in the appropriate treatment techniques
- a physiotherapist
- an osteopath
- a chiropractor.

Physiotherapy is the more traditional form of physical therapy, and usually involves the use of heat, gentle massage and exercise to help someone regain movement, strength and suppleness. Many physiotherapists are also trained in manipulation.

Osteopathy and chiropractic tend to concentrate on joint manipulation. In general, a chiropractor may use quick, gentle, specific thrusts, whereas an osteopath uses slower, more general movements. All therapists will give advice on the care and protection of the back.

In practice, however, it is doubtful whether there is much to choose between these techniques, as in all cases, the principles behind treatment are the same, and include physical activation with exercises of various types and manipulation.

Treatment for sciatica (see page 12) also involves pain-relieving tablets, rest and remobilisation, but progress is often a lot slower. Sometimes people with this particular problem have to be referred for surgery to relieve the pressure on the nerve. More information on persistent back pain is given in the next two chapters.

RECURRENT BACK PAIN

The natural history of most acute back episodes is recovery,

'These tablets have few side effects and are usually all that is necessary.'

commonly in a few days but sometimes taking a week or even a few weeks.

People with a history of backache are likely to develop further episodes in the future. Sometimes these occur as a result of an accident or an exceptional load, but for many people acute relapses may be precipitated by quite trivial physical activities. Understanding how the back works and minimising stresses on the spine, together with improvement in physical fitness, will help to prevent further recurrences.

KEY POINTS

✓ Most acute back pain is simple backache. A small proportion have sciatica and a few more severe problems

✓ Simple backache usually responds to pain relief, a short period of bed rest if necessary and early physical activation and return to work

✓ If it fails to improve, you may need to see a therapist or a specialist who may undertake further investigations and treatment

Protect your back

Some people who start off with an underlying back weakness go through repeated bouts of back pain, often because of a combination of poor posture and excessive stresses. We now know how different positions and loads affect the back and may lead to back problems, but you can teach yourself how to minimise the stresses you place on your back. These lessons are actually important for all of us, but especially for anyone who gets back pain and would like to try and prevent further attacks.

IMPROVE YOUR POSTURE

How we stand and sit is important and may greatly affect our ability to cope with back pain. Taking care over this will minimise a lot of stresses on your spine. Standing badly can stretch the spinal ligaments and cause aching and stiffness in your back.

- Stand upright with your head facing forwards, your back straight and avoid slouching

Poor   Good   Poor

Good and poor posture.

- When you're working at a bench check that it is high enough to stand with a good comfortable working posture and, in particular, that you can stand upright

Good posture   Poor posture

- A desk should be of sufficient height and with leg space so you are close enough to sit upright and work comfortably. There should be enough room beneath the work surface so that you can get close to your work without having to bend forwards and also to allow free movement of your legs and feet

Good posture   Poor posture

- Keeping still in one position for a long time is an important cause of aching and stiffness

- When sitting at a desk ensure that you can sit upright with a support in the small of your back

Good posture   Poor posture

CHECK OUT YOUR SHOES

Women who get back pain should not wear high heels. They tip the lower part of your body forwards, and you then arch your upper body backwards to compensate, so putting stress on your back. It's better to opt for shoes that don't have hard leather soles because they send shock waves up through your skeleton as your heels strike the ground and often aggravate back problems. Cushioned soles and heels or shock-absorbing insoles can reduce this and often make walking much easier. I recommend trainers as they are so comfortable and minimise these sudden shock waves.

AVOID SAGGING CHAIRS

Many chairs are poorly designed. Often the worst are low armchairs and easy chairs that look temptingly soft but hold your back in a rounded position, causing severe aching and stiffness. Perching on a stool with your back bent forwards often aggravates backache and stiffness, so avoid it if you can. You will be

Avoid sagging chairs.

Correct lumbar support.

most comfortable in an upright chair which supports your lower back, maintaining the normal slightly backward curve of the lumbar part of your spine. If necessary, you can make your own lumbar support using a small cushion or a rolled-up towel, or put a back rest or lumbar roll behind the small of your back.

COMFORT IN YOUR CAR

Backache is common in all of us who spend long periods driving. Anyone who is prone to backache can experience particular problems. In recent years car manufacturers have paid much more attention to the design of the car seat and to the driving position in order to minimise backache. However, we still find seats that are poorly designed, holding the back in a rounded position. Sitting for a long time in this posture can cause excruciating back pain. The best car seats have a built-in adjustable lumbar support. The height, seat and back angles can be altered to suit the individual driver. The foot controls should be squarely in front of your feet and not at an angle as this causes constant spine twisting. Adequate wing mirrors will help you avoid having to twist round, and power steering will lessen the strain on your spine when manoeuvring at low speeds.

Many back problems develop during lifting. Frequently this arises when load bearing is combined with bending forwards and a twist on the spine. There are some simple practical guidelines which help to protect the back and reduce the risk of back trouble.

Is the object too heavy?

The first priority when lifting is to decide whether the load is too heavy or bulky to move on your own. There are no hard and fast rules about the maximum weight that can be lifted safely. Much depends on the circumstances, the position that is required, the size, shape and weight of the object, and on your personal physical strength and health.

The strain on your spine is much greater if the object is held at arm's length rather than close to your body. Someone with back problems can carry much less than a healthy adult. On the whole men can carry heavier loads than women and young people.

The object should be held close to your body and not at arm's length. Get a firm grip with the palms of your hands and the roots of your fingers and thumbs, rather than with your fingers alone. Heavy objects should not be lifted above shoulder level as this produces tremendous strain on the spine.

Lifting objects from the floor: This is the origin of many problems. Bending forwards places great strain on the ligaments of your back and is a common cause of acute spine pain.

The right way to lift is to place your feet apart, at right angles to each other, and with the front foot pointing in the direction to which the object is to be moved. This puts you in a stable position and prevents you from twisting your back in the process of lifting and then moving off. Crouch down, bending your hips and knees but keeping your back straight. Your whole spine may be inclined

forwards but it is important to avoid bending your back. In this position, your knees are well apart and the object is positioned between them and kept close to your body. You can get a good, firm grip and the lift is performed using your leg muscles. Once you are upright, you should carry the load close to your body without twisting your back. Put it down carefully, using the same procedure in reverse.

This is known as the kinetic method of lifting. Many industries train their workers to use this technique automatically but it should be the lifting method used by everybody.

Wrong   Right

MONITOR YOUR MOVEMENTS

Bending forward and twisting movements combined with carrying a heavy load are the most likely to stress your spine and produce back problems. Avoiding this type of stress is important for all of us, but especially for anyone with a back problem.

AND SO TO BEDS

A lot of people get backache in bed. This is often because they have a poor quality mattress and base that sag under the weight of their body. Most of us sleep on our sides so sagging produces a sideways bend in the back that may lead to considerable aching and stiffness. You can largely stop this happening

A sagging mattress and too many pillows

A good quality bed

A board running the full length of the bed

Is your bed letting you down?

by sleeping on a bed that does not sag so easily. The ideal bed is one with a firm, well-sprung mattress and base, although it does not need to be hard.

In fact, it may be a mistake to buy a very firm hard bed in the belief that it is good for your back as it can be so uncomfortable that you don't sleep well. When you're choosing a bed, spend some time lying on it to ensure that it is firm but comfortable.

Unfortunately, a well-sprung, quality bed can be very expensive. An alternative which is almost as effective is to place a firm board on top of the base and underneath the mattress. It should run the full length of the bed and be thick enough not to bend under the weight of your body. Three-quarter-inch (two-centimetre) block board seems a very good choice for this purpose.

PILLOW TALK

Your whole spine should lie as straight as possible so that neither your spine nor your neck bends sideways during the night. Too many pillows put a sideways twist on your neck that will be transmitted down your back. It is usually better to use only one pillow so that your head and neck are in line with the rest of your body when lying on your side.

STAY IN SHAPE

If you are overweight, you are putting additional strain on your back, and this may mean you have a poor posture. Losing weight becomes important not only for your back, but also because it is good for your general health.

EXERCISE

Physical fitness and exercise form an important part of prevention and treatment if you are prone to back problems. We believe that exercises help to prevent back pain by increasing the ability of the trunk to cope with loads. There are many different types of exercise such as aerobics, weight-training, stretching and bending exercises (see pages 46–50). Most important is keeping fit and strengthening your spine muscles.

Some exercises can make back pain worse. If you have a back problem, it is important to be careful and to concentrate on the exercises designed for strengthening the back and stomach muscles, rather than those aimed at forcing back movements.

KEY POINTS

✓ Good posture is important for preventing backache

✓ The shoes that we wear and the chairs that we sit on can also affect our backs: avoid sagging chairs and high heels

✓ When lifting an object, follow the 'kinetic method of lifting' and avoid lifting very heavy objects

✓ Make sure that your bed has a good, firm but comfortable mattress and avoid use of too many pillows.

What causes persistent back pain?

Some people suffer persistent or chronic back pain, and need careful investigation to find out why. Once the cause is identified, a proper treatment programme can be planned.

By far the most common cause of chronic back pain is some mechanical disorder in the back. However, in a small proportion of people, pain is the result of inflammatory diseases, disorders of bone, tumours or problems in the abdomen or pelvis.

CHRONIC MECHANICAL BACK PAIN

Many people suffer persistent pain in the back which may spread into the buttock or the leg. Often, the pain is aggravated by physical activity and by certain postures. The spine is a very complicated structure and many different things

Back pain can be aggravated by your posture.

can go wrong. The following are common causes of chronic mechanical back pain.

Lumbar spondylosis or ageing changes

X-rays of the back frequently show signs of ageing changes in the intervertebral discs and facet joints. Indeed they are present in almost every older person. Although people with these ageing changes more often get backache than those without, there is only a poor correlation with the presence of symptoms. It is possible for a person to have quite severe X-ray evidence of wear and tear, and yet be symptom free. For this reason signs of wear and tear in the spine should be treated with caution. Just because you have them and also have backache does not mean that the changes are the cause of the symptoms. Nor does it mean that someone who has these changes but no backache is bound to develop back problems or become disabled in the future.

In lumbar spondylosis, the pain is felt across the low back, sometimes worse on one side than the other. The pain is worse with physical exercise and bending, and made easier by rest. However, some people tend to stiffen when lying in one position. This may be particularly noticeable first thing in the morning or after prolonged sitting in an easy chair. The pain can spread into one or other buttock and sometimes into the back of the thigh.

On examination back movements are usually limited but often this is only on certain types of movements, whereas other movements are relatively free.

Prolapsed or burst intervertebral disc

Under stress the disc may burst – usually backwards and to one side – so that it presses on a nerve, leading to pain in the back spreading down the leg. Commonly the disc was already showing marked evidence of wear and tear damage and was seriously weakened. The particular stress precipitated the development of the burst which was about to occur. When the disc prolapses, the person may develop sciatica (see page 12). The problem may persist and lead to long-term pain and disability.

The person will describe pain in the buttock usually spreading down the back or the outside of the thigh to the back of the calf and sometimes into the foot, usually the top or outer aspect. Frequently, it is accompanied by tingling or pins and needles sensations, known technically as paraesthesiae. These can be very painful and also there may be the sensation of numbness.

The examination reveals evidence that the nerve is trapped. When the leg is kept straight and lifted upwards there is a lot of pain and the movement is limited. There may be weakness of certain movements of the foot and the ankle reflex can be lost. There may be reduction in ability to feel in the area of the damaged nerve.

Hypermobility or very flexible joints and backache

Some people have remarkably flexible joints. They can bend forwards with the legs straight to place the palms of their hands flat on the ground. The joints of the arms and legs can bend to a remarkable degree. This is known as hypermobility. Many sportsmen and sportswomen, trapeze artistes and professional dancers are hypermobile because this facility enables them to undertake physical activities far beyond most of us.

Paradoxically, in later years hypermobility predisposes to development of joint symptoms. It is likely that repeated excessive movements have led to the development of wear and tear changes and overstretching of ligaments. In particular it is an important cause of back problems. It is remarkable how well back movements are preserved in these patients and sometimes they have difficulties in convincing their

Hypermobility.

doctors that there is anything wrong because their movements appear to be so good.

Inherited variations in the spine

We are all different shapes and sizes and our spines vary accordingly. Some people are born with an extra lumbar vertebra or one too few or with abnormally shaped vertebrae. These variations are usually unimportant and do not cause their owners any pain.

Spondylolisthesis

Sometimes one vertebra slips forwards on top of the one below because of a weakness in the supporting arches of the vertebral column. This is called a 'spondylolisthesis' and can cause pain because it results in overstretching of nerves or ligaments.

This slipping may be the result of failure of the supporting bones in the back of the spine to develop properly or due to wear and tear change between vertebrae.

Spinal stenosis

The nerve roots run down from the spinal cord within the column of vertebrae in the vertebral column and then emerge from the sides of the vertebral column through narrow openings (each known as a foramen, several as foramina). They then run down into the legs.

We all have spinal canals and foramina of different sizes and shapes. Some are smaller than others so that nerves that run through them are at particular risk of getting squashed.

When this affects the central canal of the vertebral column it is known as central stenosis and may lead to pain, numbness and tingling in the legs, which develop on walking and are relieved by rest. These symptoms are quite similar to the leg problems associated with a poor blood supply to the legs. The pain is also made worse by arching backwards and relieved by bending forwards.

When the narrowing affects the foramina through which the nerve roots emerge, patients may develop persistent unremitting sciatica-type pain. This is known as foraminal stenosis. Surgery to relieve these

Multiple tender areas in fibromyalgia.

types of nerve pressure can be very effective.

Fibromyalgia

People with this condition develop a range of symptoms. They experience widespread pain across the back spreading up the back of the chest into the neck and into the limbs. They often have tender points, particularly over the sacroiliac joints, the shoulder blades, the inside and outside of the elbows and knees, and elsewhere. Frequently, they have had a variety of detailed tests, but no particular abnormality can be pinpointed. Many people with fibromyalgia are very upset and depressed; they feel tired and lacking in energy. It is often difficult for doctors to decide whether the persistent pain has led to the depression or whether the depression has led them to feel pain more severely.

It may well be that the explanation lies in changes in the way pain sensations are transmitted in the spinal cord.

Many people with this condition sleep poorly and wake up in the mornings feeling unrefreshed with generalised aches and pains and stiffness. Some research suggests that this poor sleep rhythm may be responsible for the problem. People with fibromyalgia often have other problems such as irritable bowel syndrome and migraine.

OTHER CAUSES OF BACK PAIN

Although most backache is the result of mechanical disorders such as those I have described, in a small proportion of people it is a symptom of some other illness. For this reason you should always be thoroughly assessed by a doctor, particularly when back pain develops for the first time or when its nature suddenly changes. Other causes of back pain include the following.

Infection

Fortunately this is uncommon, but occasionally people with severe back problems are found to have chronic infection in the discs or elsewhere.

Ankylosing spondylitis

This is an inflammatory form of arthritis in which the effects are concentrated on the back. Sometimes it can attack the joints of the arms and legs, and occasionally other body tissues.

Most often it starts in young adults, usually men. However, women sometimes get it and it can start at any age. The initial problems appear in the joints between the sacrum and the pelvis (sacroiliac joints) and may then spread up the spine. As it advances it can cause stiffening of the back with a pronounced stoop and in severe cases the spine may end up completely rigid.

In contrast with people who have mechanical backache, those with ankylosing spondylitis usually find that their pain and stiffness are aggravated by rest and relieved by exercise. They often toss and turn in bed and wake up in the early hours of the morning with aching and stiffness. Many get up in the night and do some physical exercise in order to obtain relief. As the condition becomes more severe the aching and stiffness may last longer throughout the day.

Your doctor will examine you and probably organise blood tests and X-rays to confirm the diagnosis.

Bone disorders

The skeleton provides the scaffolding which supports the soft tissues of the body. Unlike a metal framework, bone is a living material in which the constituents are constantly being renewed. There are several types of disease which lead to weakening and deformity of the bone and may make you more prone to fractures.

• **Osteoporosis:** This is a common form of bone disease. Most often it affects women after the menopause when hormonal changes lead to weakening of bone structure, although men can and do get it too. Some people develop osteoporosis as a result of hormonal disorders such as Cushing's disease or as a complication of treatment with certain steroid drugs.

When the bone is weakened,

Osteoporosis

Normal   Osteoporotic

Thinning bones —

Thinning of the interior of bones makes them lighter and more fragile. The bones of the spine may be crushed, causing pain and loss of height.

tiny fractures occur very easily and the vertebrae become squashed. Some people experience repeated attacks of severe back pain as a result and gradually develop a stoop. The loss of height and severe bending forwards which often affects older women is usually caused by osteoporosis.

The rounded back in osteoporosis.

• **Osteomalacia:** People with this condition lack calcium and vitamin D, which can be the result of a poor diet low in dairy products, failure to absorb calcium from the bowel or lack of sunlight. Their bones become weaker, so that they are more prone to fractures and pain.

• **Paget's disease:** This condition causes the bone to suddenly start growing very quickly and affects elderly people. The new bone is abnormal and soft and may fracture easily or press on nerves and ligaments causing pain.

Tumours

Occasionally back pain may be caused by a tumour developing in the back or spreading from elsewhere. Although it is a rare cause of backache, the possibility has to be ruled out, which is why it is important to have a proper medical assessment.

Referred pain

This is the term doctors use to describe pain that you feel in your back but which actually has its origin somewhere else in your body.

Not all back pain is caused by problems in and around the spine – for example, it might be caused by disorders in the abdomen or pelvis. Stomach ulcers, gynaecological problems and some other conditions can result in pressure on nerves causing back pain. When there is some link between bouts of pain and a woman's periods, doctors will consider whether there may be a gynaecological cause. Sometimes it is not obvious that the problem is actually arising in the abdomen or pelvis.

KEY POINTS

✓ There are a number of medical conditions that cause back pain, including many mechanical disorders

✓ Back pain can also be a symptom of some other illness, such as inflammation, infection, bone disorders, referred pain, etc.

✓ Ageing changes can cause back problems in elderly people

✓ In women after the menopause, osteoporosis can cause back pain and bending of the spine

Treating persistent back pain

FIRST STEP – GETTING A DIAGNOSIS

Your medical history

For your doctor, the most important part of assessing your back problem is finding out from you exactly how the pain started and what has happened since, together with other medical features. You will then have a physical examination. That may well be all that is necessary.

Blood tests

As we have seen, most backaches have a mechanical cause, so the results of blood tests are normal. However, such tests are useful when investigating possible inflammatory and other causes of back pain. In particular ankylosing spondylitis (see page 39) is associated with a certain white blood cell type known as HLA-B27.

If this is not present when your blood test results come back, you are very unlikely to have this condition. The opposite is not the case, however, as this white cell type is found in about eight per cent of healthy people who do not have ankylosing spondylitis.

X-rays

Vast numbers of spine X-rays are taken but the majority are unnecessary. The only people who really need them are those with severe back pain that has failed to get better with simple treatment and those with complicated problems. Unnecessary X-rays should be avoided as each involves some, albeit slight, exposure to radiation.

Radiculography

When we look at X-rays of the spine we are actually studying shadows of

CT scan.

the bones. This means we cannot see the soft tissues such as the nerves and discs within the spine. In a radiculogram (myelogram), dye that is opaque to X-rays is injected into the spinal column. When a disc has burst the column of dye will be indented so that the exact location of the damaged disc can be identified on the X-ray.

CT scans

CT stands for computed tomography. CT scans enable doctors to use X-rays to obtain a clearer view of the internal structures of the vertebral column. In particular the inner outlines of the bony structures can be examined and some details of the discs can be seen.

MRI scans

MRI stands for magnetic resonance imaging and is the latest scanning technique. It involves the use of very strong magnetic fields rather than X-rays, and is particularly good for studying the nerves, ligaments and discs within the bony structures.

CT and MRI scans are gradually becoming more widely available. However, it's not always clear who can really benefit from being scanned in these ways. As with

MRI scan.

X-rays of the back, the changes that they reveal often correlate poorly with symptoms.

TREATMENT

How chronic back pain is treated depends on whether it is caused by mechanical problems – the most common kind – or by some other disorder.

Caring for your back

Physical activity is good for people with chronic back problems. You should try to keep active and to exercise, although you do need to take some sensible precautions. You have to be careful, for example, to avoid over-stressing your back and to be aware of your posture when standing, sitting and lifting. Lifting heavy loads is not a job for you.

Physiotherapy

Views on treatment have changed dramatically in the last few years. We now believe the principal role of the physiotherapist is to get you mobile again and restore you to normal levels of activity as soon as possible. It is important that you be referred to a physiotherapist if your back problem has lasted more than a few weeks and is in danger of becoming chronic.

The physiotherapist will teach you how your back works, what can go wrong, how to protect the back against excessive stresses and teach you exercises aimed at restoring your mobility so you can start to function normally again.

The exercise programme will normally be tailored to your individual needs, but will include

Teaching a patient about the spine and back problems.

ones to strengthen your back and abdominal muscles, together with pelvic tilt exercises.

Sometimes, the physiotherapist will apply various forms of heat such as an infrared lamp or short-wave diathermy, or of cold with ice packs or cooling aerosol sprays, ultrasound or massage. Such treatments do not cure the long-term problem but can be extremely soothing and relaxing. Their special value is often as a preliminary to other forms of treatment such as exercises, which otherwise would be very painful.

Traction, like many of the treatments of back pain, has been used since ancient times. You lie on a special traction table with one harness around your lower chest, another round your pelvis and the two halves of your body are gently pulled apart. The idea is to stretch damaged joints and relieve pressure on damaged nerves. It helps at the time but its long-term value is doubtful and its use is becoming restricted. It is not worth rushing out to buy any of the expensive gadgets available on the market for home traction.

Exercises

There are many different types of exercise for people with chronic back pain, and the choice depends very much on the nature of your particular problem. Some exercises may help one type of backache but make another worse so be careful when planning your own exercise programme.

You should discuss these first with your physiotherapist. The various types of exercise include those already described, aimed at strengthening the back and abdominal muscles (known as isometric exercises), and those that improve movements of the back. It is important to avoid any exercises that make the pain suddenly worse. It is better to undertake a specific amount of exercise which is gradually increased each day.

An exercise programme

A simple and safe programme of exercises should be undertaken in a graded and gradually increasing fashion. Initially do the following exercises once or twice and then gradually increase up to six times each day as your back allows.

For many people, other types of exercise are required, but these should be performed only under the guidance of a physio-therapist because certain exercises can make some patients worse. Much depends upon the particular problems in each individual case.

1 Lie flat on your back on the floor. Keep the legs straight and lift each heel in turn, just off the floor. Repeat.

2 Lie flat on your back on the floor with a pillow under your head. Fold your arms. Lift your head and shoulders just off the floor and then lie flat and relax. Repeat.

3 Lie flat on your back on the floor. Tense your stomach muscles and flatten the small of your back onto the floor, then relax. Repeat.

If any of these exercises aggravate the back pain, then they should not be performed.

4 Lie flat on your back. Reach down the side of one thigh towards the knee. Straighten up and repeat to the other side. Repeat.

Seen from above.

5 Lie flat on your back on the floor. Bend your knees so that your feet are flat on the ground, then lift your bottom in the air by tightening the stomach muscles, keeping the back straight. Repeat.

If any of these exercises aggravate the back pain, then they should not be performed.

6 Lie on your stomach on the floor, then do press-ups with your hands, but keeping your back straight. Repeat.

7 Kneel on all fours. Arch and hollow your back. Then flatten your back. Repeat.

If any of these exercises aggravate the back pain, then they should not be performed.

8 Stand with your back against the wall. Tighten the tummy muscles so that your back flattens against the wall. Then restore the normal hollow and repeat.

8a

8b

If any of these exercises aggravate the back pain, then they should not be performed.

Sport

Sportsmen should keep active and return to sport as soon as possible after a bout of severe pain. The safest options are walking, swimming and cycling. Contact sports such as rugby are risky as sudden, unexpected and forceful move-

ments of the back can undo several weeks of gradual improvement.

Mobilisation and manipulation

If back pain is caused by mechanical displacement of one of the joints or discs then it should be possible to put things right by manipulation of

Swim on your tummy or on your back, whichever is
most comfortable.

the spine. This is the theory underlying the various techniques of mobilisation and manipulation. There is wide variety in the techniques practised by physiotherapists, osteopaths, chiropractors, physicians and orthopaedic surgeons.

Some manipulators apply forces directly to the vertebrae in the spine whereas others use the shoulders and pelvis as levers. There is no agreement on the problems for which manipulation is useful, when the different types of manipulation should be used and the relative usefulness of these treatments by the various practitioners. Manipulation can hasten your recovery from an acute episode of back pain but it is doubtful whether it provides real benefit for chronic back pain.

In general manipulation appears to be safe, although a few people find that it makes their back problems worse. There is a very small risk of nerve damage when manipulation is performed under anaesthetic.

MEDICINES AND TABLETS

The main purpose of drugs is to relieve pain. The two main types used are pure pain relievers known as analgesics and those – known as anti-inflammatory drugs – which also control inflammation in the area of damage. The character of the back problem is often helpful in indicating which type of drug will be most effective.

Painkillers

Paracetamol is the most commonly used painkiller. You can take up to six or eight 500 milligram tablets a day and it is very safe provided you don't exceed this dose. You can buy paracetamol by itself or combined with other drugs such as codeine from chemists without a doctor's prescription. There are several stronger analgesics such as dextropropoxyphene and dihydrocodeine which are often combined with paracetamol, but these are only available on prescription.

Anti-inflammatory drugs

You'll find these particularly helpful if you have a lot of stiffness in bed and when you wake up in the morning. Their main role is to reduce inflammation, but they are effective pain killers as well. Aspirin was the first anti-inflammatory drug but it can cause indigestion and abdominal upsets, and larger doses may give you ringing noises in your ears and interfere with your hearing. Ibuprofen is available over the counter in pharmacies and seems to produce far fewer problems.

There are alternative anti-inflammatory drugs available on prescription, such as naproxen, diclofenac, piroxicam, ketoprofen and many others. These are generally taken in tablet form. A lot of research has gone into producing newer versions that need only be taken once or twice a day rather than every few hours – an obvious advantage. All the anti-inflammatory drugs can cause abdominal upsets, so you may be prescribed an anti-ulcer treatment to take at the same time. Alternatively, if the anti-inflammatory tablets upset your system too much, your doctor can prescribe suppositories instead.

Muscle relaxants

If you are one of those people who develop quite severe spasm of the back muscles, which is very painful, you may find that muscle relaxant tablets are a help.

Anti-epileptic drugs

Neuralgic pains are sudden electric shock sensations shooting from the back down the leg, often accompanied by painful tingling and numbness. These symptoms seem to result from over-sensitivity of the damaged nerves. People with epilepsy have over-sensitive brain cells which fire off in an uncontrolled way, causing them to have seizures (or fits). The same drugs which are used to counter that problem can also be effective in relieving neuralgic pain.

Tricyclic antidepressants

Some people who have chronic back problems develop widespread pain and often their skin becomes hypersensitive so that it is tender to even light pressure. Alteration in the pain-processing system in the central nervous system probably underlies this. This type of pain is not helped by conventional pain-relieving tablets. There may be similar biochemical changes in the central nervous systems of people who are clinically depressed, and the drugs used for treating depression such as amitriptyline can also be effective for treating this kind of pain.

Injections

Injections can be very helpful for certain types of back pain. They take a number of different forms depending upon the precise nature of the problem.

• **For tender spots:** Some people with back problems have one or two very localised tender areas in their back – perhaps in the superficial tissues, in the ligaments connecting the vertebrae, the sacroiliac joints or elsewhere. Your doctor can identify the painful areas by feeling your back carefully while you are lying flat in a relaxed position. The tender spots may then be treated with an injection of a small amount of local anaesthetic and a powerful steroid, such as cortisone. Steroids also have long-lasting anti-inflammatory action. After the injection you will usually be pain free for two to three hours due to the anaesthetic, then the pain may return for 24 hours or so. However, after that period, some people find that their pain diminishes dramatically. How long this relief lasts varies considerably from one person to another, but for many it is long lasting. Cortisone used in this way does not cause the adverse effects that may develop when it is taken regularly by mouth.

• **Facet joint injections:** Sometimes the problem arises in the facet joints at the back of the spine, and this can also be treated by means of an injection using a fine needle. It is usually done under X-ray guidance so that the injection can be positioned in precisely the right place in the joint.

• **Epidural injections:** An epidural injection is given into the spine around the linings surrounding the spinal cord and nerve roots. Local anaesthetic with a small amount of a cortisone-like drug is injected. You may be offered this if you have sciatica that has improved after a severe attack but has not cleared up completely.

OTHER TREATMENTS

Acupuncture

Back pain can be very difficult to control. Sometimes, the symptoms are relieved by blocking the passage of nerve impulses up the spine to the brain.

Acupuncture was first developed in China between 2,000 and 3,000 years ago. It was thought to work by altering the balance between the two opposing life forces known as Yin and Yang. Acupuncture is often used in Western medicine today. We now know that it stimulates the release of natural chemicals known as endorphins and enkephalins within the brain and spinal cord which can block the passage of the pain sensations. Sterile needles are inserted through the skin and then rotated to produce stimulation. Some acupuncturists use the traditional Chinese acupuncture sites but for many this is out of custom rather than belief.

Acupuncture does not work on everybody. Some people respond well, others derive only short-term

Needle being rotated

Acupuncture.

benefit and need repeated treatment, and for some acupuncture makes no difference at all.

Transcutaneous electrical nerve stimulation (TENS)

The problem with acupuncture is that inserting needles through the skin and applying stimulation is a highly skilled technique and you have to attend a special clinic to have it done. TENS, on the other hand, is a treatment which you can give yourself in your own home. You fix electric pads coated with a special electrical conducting jelly to the skin of your back. These are then connected to a battery and stimulator which you wear on your belt.

When you switch the gadget on, multiple tiny pulses of electricity stimulate your skin, and you can adjust the strength, frequency and length of time of each impulse to suit yourself. The electrical stimulation feels like a tiny pricking sensation in your skin. It acts in a similar way to acupuncture by stimulating nerves and releases substances in the brain and spinal cord that block the sensation of back pain.

This technique is useful for someone with chronic back pain who can switch on the stimulator whenever he or she needs it. TENS does not help everybody but can be remarkably successful for some.

The TENS apparatus.

Corsets

The lumbar support or corset consists of a firm body belt stretching from the rib cage to the pelvis with strengtheners behind which may be flat steel strips moulded to the shape of the back. Wearing one limits your back movements and increases the pressure within your abdomen and therefore may relieve back pain. Unfortunately, wearing a corset for a long time can lead to permanent back stiffness and in the long run many corsets do as much harm as good. We now believe that, for most people, the aim should be to restore movements to the back as soon as possible, which is why corsets are now used only rarely.

SURGERY

It is estimated that only about one operation is needed for every 2,000 attacks of back pain. Surgery should only be considered if your symptoms have not responded to other treatment, if you have severe and persisting pain, and if your problem is of the type likely to improve after an operation. This means that surgery is unlikely to be considered as soon as an attack of back pain develops. Rather, other types of treatment will be tried first, and most people recover without the need for an operation. If you reach the point where an operation is being considered, your surgeon will arrange for detailed investigations to be performed.

Only certain types of back problems are likely to respond well to surgery. In particular there are very good results for those who have severe sciatic pain in the leg. About 80 to 90 per cent of people are very pleased with the results. On the other hand, the success rate is not nearly as good for those whose main problem is pain in the back itself.

What operation?

There are several different types of back operation. The most common is to remove a prolapsed disc – usually this is the disc between the fourth and fifth lumbar vertebrae or between the fifth lumbar vertebra and the sacrum. In order to prevent any recurrence, the whole disc is usually removed and not just the burst area. In some cases the main problem is pressure on the nerve roots from the bone of the vertebral column. The surgeon will aim to relieve this by taking away bone to create more space. Sometimes there is excessive movement between the bones of the vertebral column. The surgeon may decide to fix the vertebrae together. This is known as a spinal fusion.

Convalescence

After surgery you will probably start to get up and walk within a few days. Often you have to wear a lumbar support for a few weeks but you may well get back to light work within a month or two. It will be several months before you can consider doing any heavy manual work. You should always ask your surgeon before undertaking activities likely to cause excessive loads on your spine.

Intensive rehabilitation

A small proportion of people with chronic back pain develop very severe symptoms and become very disabled. There are a number of reasons for this, including not only the mechanical forms of damage around the spine, but also scarring which may develop around the nerve roots. This is known as arachnoiditis. There may be other changes which may occur within the central nervous system itself, and the whole problem is often exacerbated by depression and anxiety. Unfortunately, this type of back pain can be very difficult to treat. People in this situation will need a careful and sympathetic assessment which will include not only analysis of the physical problem but also of their reactions to it.

The next stage is to design an intensive rehabilitation programme tailored to the requirements of each individual, which aims not only to restore physical function but also to help the person concerned to cope with the problem and to lead a more normal life. This type of treatment can be very effective for the most severely disabled back sufferers. Unfortunately the availability of this type of programme, such as the one that we run in the Manchester and Salford Back Pain Centre, is extremely limited and currently is provided at very few centres in Britain. It is hoped that these facilities will become more widely available before too long.

KEY POINTS

✓ The clinical examination is the most important part of assessment. The imaging tests are a useful supplement in appropriate cases

✓ The back sufferer should understand how the back works, what goes wrong and why various types of treatment are used

✓ Exercise is good for the back but sudden forceful movements should be avoided

✓ The choice of tablets is related to the clinical problem. Most patients will be controlled by a simple pain killer such as paracetamol or anti-inflammatory drugs such as ibuprofen

✓ Surgery is only rarely necessary. On the whole it works a lot better for sciatic pain in the leg than for back pain alone

✓ Intensive rehabilitation programmes are effective for people with severe chronic back problems

Useful addresses

There are several national societies which are concerned with the welfare of people with back pain and with raising funds for research for better methods of diagnosis and treatment. Several of these organisations produce helpful booklets which provide useful factual information.

The Arthritis and Rheumatism Council
I Copeman House
St Mary's Court, St Mary's Gate
Chesterfield
Derbyshire S41 7TD
Tel: 01246 558033

This charity finances an extensive programme of research and education in a wide range of arthritis and rheumatism problems including back pain. It provides useful booklets explaining the various back problems and ways of coping with them.

Arthritis Care
18 Stephenson Way
London NW1 2HD
Tel: 0171 916 1500

This charity provides information and advice for those who are disabled by all forms of arthritis and back pain. In particular it runs holiday hotels for people disabled with arthritis and publishes a quarterly newsletter, *Arthritis News*, which is sent to all members.

National Ankylosing Spondylitis Society
3 Grosvenor Crescent
London SW1X 7ER
Tel (answerphone): 0171 235 9585

This charity is for patients with ankylosing spondylitis, their families and friends, and doctors and research workers concerned with this problem. It provides practical advice and help, and holds open meetings for members. It publishes a useful handbook, a cassette tape of physiotherapy exercises, a twice-yearly journal and other publications.

National Back Pain Association
16 Elmtree Road
Teddington
Middlesex TW11 8ST
Tel: 0181 977 5474

This charity has local branches throughout the country with regular meetings to disseminate information and advice for people with back pain. Its mission is to fund patient-oriented scientific research into the causes and treatment of back pain, to educate people to use their bodies sensibly and so reduce the incidence of back pain, and to form and support branches through which sufferers and those who care for them may receive information, advice and mutual help.

National Osteoporosis Society
PO Box 10
Radstock
Bath BA3 3YB
Tel: 01761 471771

This is a charitable organisation which provides advice and support for people with osteoporosis and seeks to improve general awareness and sponsor research into this problem.

The Spinal Injuries Association
76 St James' Lane
London N10 3DF
Tel: 0181 444 2121

This charity is for spinal cord injury people, their families and friends. It offers a range of services for paraplegics and tetraplegics. It publishes a regular newsletter with useful practical advice and help.

FURTHER READING
A more detailed account of back problems and their treatment can be found in *Back Pain: The Facts* by MIV Jayson, Oxford University Press, 1992.

Index

The National Back Pain Association

A registered medical charity, working to help people with back problems – we :

- Fund research

- Provide educational literature to help people with back problems

- Run a countrywide network of self help branches for chronic sufferers

- Operate a specialist nurse helpline for members and their families

- Offer a new care & repair scheme based on safe exercise. BACKWATCHERS is for people with recurring back problems and is available for use in professional settings

Further information from: National Back Pain Association
16 Elmtree Road, Teddington, Middx TW11 8ST
Tel: 0181–977 5474   Fax: 0181–943 5318
Send £2.50 for an information pack to this address

Reg. Charity No. 256751

PHYSIOTHERAPY
DENTAL, OPTICAL
Plus 17 more 'Super' Health Care Cash Benefits

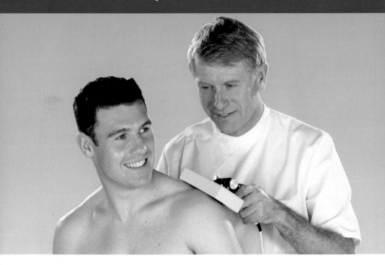

HSA SuperPlan leads the way in family health care cash plans. One payment covers all the family for **20** generous health care CASH benefits.
No increase in premiums with age.

FROM AROUND
21p TO **£1.66**
A DAY

CALL FREE **0800 150 150**
QUOTING REFERENCE MK 0209 FOR DETAILS

HSA Healthcare, Hambleden House, ANDOVER, Hants. SP10 1LQ.
or 28 Stafford Street, EDINBURGH EH3 7BD.